LOVE IS FISHY

31 Delicious Fish Recipes Told Through a Love Story

by

Duc Vuong, M.D.

ISBN-13: 978-0692973936

ISBN-10: 0692973931

Published by HappyStance Publishing.

Interior formatting and cover design by Tony Loton of LOTONtech Limited, www.lotontech.com.

www.SleeveAcademy.com

For My Patients,

who inspire me every day with their courage.

INTRODUCTION

Sometimes you find love where you least expect it. Your new life can be waiting behind any corner. It's up to you to look up.

It's hard to maintain a healthy lifestyle while balancing your career and personal life. For most people, it's nearly impossible. But sometimes, you'll find that if you take care of yourself, the world has a way of taking care of you. After all, it's hard to love others unless you love yourself first.

Which brings us to our story. It's a love story, but it's more than that. It's the story of family, friends and coming together over good food to share experiences both good and bad. It's a story told through vignettes and recipes, full of the spice of life. And it starts with one man's desire to follow a heart-healthy diet that includes delicious yet simple-to-prepare fish dishes.

Our hero, Binh, is a hard-working but shy accountant, whose family is from Vietnam. Though kind-hearted and modestly successful in life, love has always eluded him. So he decides to learn a new skill that might come in handy for a dating life.

CONTENTS

CHAPTER 1 – SALMON SEEKING WOMAN

The shops are crowded. It's a sunny Friday afternoon in March--a rare and fortunate day that no one should let go to waste. Everyone is out and about, shopping for picnics, picking up the next week's groceries, preparing for a big Sunday meal. Shoppers flit from aisle to aisle like bees sipping nectar from the tulips.

A lanky young man is holding his shopping basket close to his body, trying to make himself as small as possible so as to not become an obstacle for other shoppers. He sticks to the outside of the shop--avoiding the processed foods and fatty snacks stocked on the shelves in the interior of the brightly lit store. He favors fresh, green vegetables, fruits, lean meats and fish that are high in Omega-3 fats. His one weakness are macaroons, and he picks up a small box for a treat.

As he makes his way through the busy produce section, he takes in the festival of colors. The bright, vivid oranges, reds and yellows in the fruit stand. The earthy browns and deep shades of emerald of the root vegetables and leafy greens. He makes his selections--a few sweet potatoes, some spinach, a crown of broccoli, a bunch of bananas and a bag of mandarin oranges--and proceeds past the pre-packed lunch meats to the butcher's counter.

"Good morning, Binh, what can I do for you today?" the plump, older man behind the counter cheerfully asks.

Binh looks over the selection. His gentle, almond shaped eyes fall on the wild caught salmon, glistening and ruby red on its bed of crushed ice. "That salmon looks great."

"Ah, yes, nice choice. It also happens to be on sale today. There was a mix up with the ordering, and we have a surplus. How much would you like?"

"I'll take a pound, please. There's so much I can do with a nice piece of fish like this!"

"Right you are, Binh. I'll get that for you right away." The ruddy butcher removes a large fillet from the sparkling fish case and turns to weigh and cut the salmon.

As the the butcher works, Binh catches the scent of a delicate, magnolia laced perfume. He turns, trying to be as inconspicuous as possible. But when he sees the source of the intoxicating scent, he is stunned into rigid stillness.

That's the most beautiful woman I've ever seen, he thought. And then, I better stop gawking before she notices me.

The most beautiful woman Binh had ever seen is fumbling with her purse, searching the expansive bag for something. She doesn't notice Binh's dumbfounded stare or his flushed, blushing cheeks.

"Here you go, sir," the butcher says, breaking Binh's concentration on the fair skinned, rosy lipped, delicate flower of a woman, single-mindedly digging through her belongings. Her hand emerges from the bag, clasping a crinkled shopping list. She looks up, and Binh whips around to face the cheery man behind the counter.

Binh accepts the package, wrapped twice in waxy, brown paper, and manages a mumbled "thank you." He sheepishly slinks away from the counter, glancing behind him every few seconds as he goes for just one more glimpse of the astoundingly beautiful mystery woman.

The butcher's jovial greeting can be heard from quite a few feet away, "Nice to see you again, Tam. Can I interest you in today's catch?"

Binh inhales deeply once he's out of earshot and tries to commit to memory the scent of her enticing perfume. So her name is Tam, he thinks, Tam. What a perfect name. Binh considers going back to the counter, pretending he'd forgotten something, so he could try to talk to her. The very thought makes his brow sweat. Or I could just ask the butcher about her. He knows everyone in the neighborhood. Is that too weird? What if he tells her I asked about her?

Binh weighs his options and decides talking to the butcher is the path least likely to induce a heart attack. He ducks into the cereal aisle, feigning like he's browsing the whole grain options. When he hears the soft clack of Tam's heels, Binh pokes his head out to make sure the coast, and the counter, are clear. Taking a deep, jagged breath, he abandons the bran flakes and granola cereals and reapproaches the fish counter.

"Hi again, Binh! Did you forget something?" the butcher booms.

"No. No, no..." Binh stammers, shrinking at the butcher's resounding voice, hoping beyond hope that Tam couldn't hear what he was about to ask. "I..." Binh starts. He takes another deep breath and starts again. "I was hoping you could do me a small kindness and not think it's too weird but that girl who was just here. I think her name is Tam. Do you know anything about her?"

The jovial butcher chuckles, and his entire body shakes with the gesture. "Ah, young love," he smiles with a sparkle in his eyes. "Yes, you are right. Her name is Tam. Her father is a banker in the city, and her mother sadly passed away many years ago." The butcher pauses for a moment, somber and seemingly lost in thought. "I believe she is studying art history or museum curating, or...something to do with the fine arts at the University."

Binh hesitates. "But..." he squeaks out. "But is she single?"

*   *   *

Binh totes his brown paper grocery bag up the five flights of stairs to his loft style apartment. He shifts his weight, secures the bag between his hip and the crux of his arm, and slides his key into the lock. The door opens with a small click and a long, pronounced creak.

Before he can set his bag on the dark granite counters in his open galley kitchen, his orange tabby, Ginger, nuzzles his shin and weaves between his legs, purring softly and vocalizing her desire to be fed.

"Hey there kitty," Binh says as he carefully makes his way to the counter and deposits his bag next to the built-in gas range. "Do you smell that salmon? That's for people. You can have kitty kibble." Binh feeds Ginger first, before returning to the kitchen to prepare his own meal.

Selecting the salmon and broccoli for tonight's dinner, Binh stores the rest of his groceries and removes a cast iron skillet, stock pot and bamboo steamer from the cupboard.

Finally, time to eat. What a day. He unwraps the wild-caught salmon, and its ruby red hue reminds him of Tam's shade of lipstick.

HERO RECIPE – BINH'S PAN SEARED SALMON

Makes 3-4 servings

<u>Ingredients</u>

1 pound wild-caught salmon fillet, skin-on
2 tbsp peanut oil or olive oil
Salt
Lemon

<u>Method</u>

Start with a fresh, ruby red fillet. We will start our cooking with the simplest of recipes.

Sprinkle the fish with salt and pepper.

Heat the oil in a cast iron skillet over medium high heat. There should just be just enough oil to cover the bottom of the pan and prevent the fish from sticking. We're searing, not frying.

Place the fish skin down into the pan and allow it to sear for about 3 minutes. Do not try to move the fish. Once the skin has crisped, you can start to move it with a fish spatula. Flip it over for 1-2 minutes until desired doneness.

Leave center slightly translucent. The fish will continue to cook once removed.

Squeeze fresh lemon juice over the fillet and garnish with lemon slices and dill.

Honey Glazed Salmon

Makes 4 servings

<u>Ingredients</u>

1 lb salmon, cut into 4 fillets
4 tbsp all purpose flour
4 tbsp honey
2 tbsp olive oil
Salt and pepper to taste
Zest of 1 lime

<u>Method</u>

Preheat oven to 400° F.

Season both sides of salmon with salt and pepper. Dredge each fillet in flour and drizzle with honey.

Heat olive oil over medium-high heat in an oven-proof skillet. When oil is hot, sear salmon until golden brown on both sides--about 2 minutes per side.

Place skillet and salmon in the preheated oven until cooked through--about 6-8 minutes. Serve immediately with lime zest.

Salmon Burgers

Makes 2 servings

<u>Ingredients</u>

¾ pound salmon, skinless & boneless
1 tsp Dijon mustard
1 shallot, peeled and chopped
¼ cup coarse breadcrumbs
½ tbsp capers, drained
1 tbsp olive oil Salt and pepper Lemon wedges

For the burger:Brioche bun

> *Fresh spinach leaves*

Tabasco aioli:

> *2 tbsp lite mayonnaise*
> *1 tbsp lemon juice*
> *1 tbsp Tabasco*

<u>Method</u>

Cut the salmon into chunks. Place about ¼ of the fish in a food processor or blender with the Dijon mustard and mix until pasty. You may need to stop and scrape down the sides from time to time.

Add the rest of the salmon and shallots. Pulse the mixture until well combined. The largest pieces within the mixture should be no larger than a quarter inch. Do not over mix.

Transfer the mixture to a large bowl. Mix in the capers, breadcrumbs, salt and pepper by hand, then form into patties.

Heat the olive oil on medium heat. Cook the burgers for 2-3 minutes per side, turning once. Serve on a brioche bun with lemon wedges, spinach and Tabasco aioli.

For The Aioli:

Whisk together 2 tbsp lite mayonnaise, 1 tbsp lemon juice and 1 tbsp Tabasco. Chill until ready to use.

SALMON SALAD

Makes 2 servings
A great way to use leftover salmon is to make a healthy, fresh salad.

Ingredients

3 cups baby spinach, washed and dried
½ avocado, cubed
1 tbsp toasted walnuts, chopped
1 tbsp toasted sunflower seeds
1 tbsp dried cranberries
olive oil
salt and pepper
1 ½ tbsp balsamic vinaigrette

Method

To make vinaigrette, mix 1/2 balsamic vinegar with ½ olive oil. Salt and pepper to taste. You can also use your favorite premade brand.

Toss spinach with vinaigrette in a large bowl. Half the spinach and place on two plates. Top with leftover salmon and remaining ingredients. Simple, easy, delicious and good for you!

CHAPTER 2 – IN AND TROUT OF LOVE

The vibration on his bedside table wakes Binh from a light sleep. He is dreaming of Tam, picnicking by the lake. His hand grazed hers. He leaned in for a kiss--and then his eyes flutter open, blinking against the dim early morning light. His right hand shoots out blindly and retrieves his vibrating phone from its dock on the night stand. Binh licks his lips and sighs. The phone reads 5:47 AM. On a Saturday.

"Hello?" Binh tries to disguise his annoyance. And then, his heart beats faster as he rouses and realizes something might be wrong. Why else would someone call this early?

"Binh. Hi. It's me, Kat. I know it's early or late, or...I don't know. I haven't slept in 3 days. I just, I need a friend right now, okay? She's gone..." the voice on the phone blurts and sputters.

Binh struggles to piece it all together in his drowsy stupor. He wishes he were still dreaming of Tam. "Wait. What? Who's gone? Kat? Are you okay?"

"I think so. I don't know. I mean, I'm not in physical pain. I feel like I'm dying, but nothing's broken, other than my heart. She left me, man. Amy left me. It's just me, myself and no Amy, man. I don't know what to do. My life is over." Kat has always had a flair for the dramatic.

Sensing that her owner is awake, Ginger bounds onto the bed and gently caresses Binh's chin with the top of her head. Well, I guess I'm up now, Binh thinks, resigning himself to an early start this morning.

Kat is still talking, "...and I just thought, I don't know. I don't know what to think. Everything is terrible."

"Kat. It's early. I want to sleep. But I also want to help you. What can I do? Do you want to come over this afternoon and grill out? Or we could hit the pubs, blow off some steam?"

"Yeah, no. Grilling out sounds good. I don't want to go out. I've been drinking too much since Amy left, anyway. And seeing other girls just makes me think of her, and seeing other couples just makes me angry. Yeah. I should sleep, too. I'll try to get some rest and see you at yours around, what? Noon?"

"Noon sounds great, Kat. Now get some sleep. You're not thinking straight."
"Yeah. Yeah. See you soon, man."

Binh's vision is obscured by a fluffy orange blur. "Well, hello, Ginger. I guess it's time to get up. Maybe we can have some breakfast and both take a little cat nap." Binh strokes his tabby. Her tail traces an S in the grey morning glow.

*   *   *

There's a lot to be done before Kat arrives. Binh has had a busy week at work. He's an accountant, and it is tax season. So, his apartment is not in the best of shape. There's a courtyard in his building with a communal grill, picnic tables and gazebo, but Kat will likely want to talk in private, away from nosy neighbors and gossips.

Luckily, the cozy size of Binh's loft makes cleaning and washing up less of a challenge. He makes his full-sized bed, pulling the down comforter and grey duvet over his pillows and off-white sheets, and slides out a simple shoji screen to separate his sleeping area from the rest of the loft.

His bedroom nook opens into a large living space, sparsely decorated but furnished with a keen eye for aesthetic. The exposed ductwork creates interesting shadows and highlights on the ceiling, amid the minimalist track lighting. To the left, a large, bay window looks out over the small, but vibrant, downtown area where Binh lives.

In the center of the living area, a short pile chevron area rug in buttercream and heather protects the chestnut hardwood floors. Two charcoal modular armchairs sit cater-cornered, in front of a petite fireplace and mantle, an end table with a modest lamp between them.

To the right of the fireplace, a small cafe table and integrated breakfast bar comprise the dining area that abuts the galley kitchen.

Binh is wrapping up some paperwork in an armchair, Ginger in his lap and his laptop on the end table, when Kat arrives.

She bursts in without knocking. That has always been Kat's way. Her long, unkempt hair follows behind her, bringing with it the scent of earth and rose water. She stands at five-foot flat, but manages to take up the whole room when she enters.

"Well, she's gone." Kat begins, without hesitation. "I thought we could work it out, so I didn't take it seriously. Y'know, we have these fights. She goes to her mom's, I stay and take care of the dogs. But this time is really it. Amy is done with me." She flops into the armchair adjacent to where Binh is sitting.

"Hi, Kat." Binh says.

"God. I'm so rude. How are you? What's going on in your life?" Kat shifts in her chair to look directly at Binh.

"Taxes, mostly," Binh laughs dryly. "And this other thing. Well, it's not really a thing. It's more like a, I dunno, a..."

"Oooh, tell me!" Kat interrupts.

"I don't know if it's really the right time..."

"Oh, just tell me. It will help get my mind off Amy."

"Okay, well. I saw a girl in the market. And I'm trying to find her. I've been back to the fish counter 3 times this week, hoping to run into her again. We're having trout tonight, on a related note."

"Haha! What do you know about her? Do you even know her name? This is so like you, Binh." "Her name is Tam. Her father is a banker, and she studies some kind of art at the University. But that's all I've got. Other than the fish counter thing. I feel great tho--all the lean fish I've been eating."

"Oh. Em. Gee. Tam? There's a Tam in my spin class!" Kat whips out her smartphone. "Here. I'll show you and you can tell me if it's her."

Kat's thumbs fly over the screen and a picture of a smiling young girl appears. Binh's heart is in his throat. His pulse races and his palms feel sweaty. Surely it can't be this easy to find her. The city's not that small.

"Is this her?" Kat shoves the phone a little too close to Binh's face in her excitement.

"Well, let me see." Binh takes the phone and inspects it. His shoulders slump.

"No. It's not her." "Damn," Kat sighs. "Well, now we're in the same boat, it seems. But y'know what will solve our lady troubles? Food. Let's grill."

HERO RECIPE: PLANK GRILLED RAINBOW TROUT

Makes 3-4 servings
Another easy recipe for our Hero, another easy recipe for you.

Ingredients

Charcoal or gas grill
Cedar wood plank
Rainbow trout fillets
Butter, room temperature
Salt & pepper

Method

Soak a cedar wood grilling plank in water, completely submerged, for at least an hour.

Heat the grill to 300ºF. Place the plank on the grill and allow to sit for 5 minutes.

Flip the wood and oil or butter the cooking surface.

Place the trout on the cedar plank. Brush with soft butter and season with salt and pepper.

Allow to cook, with the grill lid open, until done. Trout fillets are typically thin, and will cook quickly.

BLACKENED TROUT

Makes 6 servings

Note* This dish will smoke. Have windows and doors open.

Ingredients

1 tbsp paprika
2 tsp dry mustard
1 tsp cayenne
1 tsp ground cumin
1 tsp black pepper
1 tsp white pepper
1 tsp dried thyme
1 tsp salt
1 cup unsalted butter, melted
6 4oz trout fillets

Method

Mix dry ingredients together in a small bowl and set aside. Heat a cast iron skillet over high heat for about 10 minutes.

Pour ¾ cup of melted butter into a shallow dish. Dredge each fillet. Sprinkle with spice mixture and pat gently into the fish.

Place fillets in the hot pan. Avoid crowding and work in batches if you need. Carefully spoon about 1 tsp butter over each fillet and cook until fish has a charred appearance, or about 2 minutes.

Flip and repeat.

TROUT CASSEROLE

Makes 4 servings

This healthy twist on casserole replaces a béchamel sauce with a cauliflower puree. It's also a great way to repurpose trout leftovers.

Ingredients

1 small onion, chopped
2 cloves garlic, minced
½ tsp sea salt
½ tsp black pepper
1 small cauliflower, roughly chopped
1 cup light chicken stock
¼ cup clarified butter
1 tbsp Dijon mustard
1 lb. leftover cooked trout
½ lb Brussel sprouts
¼ lb roasted butternut squash
¼ cup chopped pistachio
1-2 tbsp extra virgin olive oil

Method

Preheat oven to 375ºF.

Cook onion, garlic, salt and pepper over medium heat in a medium saucepan until fragrant. Add the cauliflower and cook for an additional 2 minutes or so.

Pour in the chicken stock and cover. Bring to a low boil and simmer until the cauliflower is tender, about 6 minutes.

Ladle the cauliflower mixture into a blender. Combine with clarified butter and Dijon mustard. Blend on high until silky. Set aside.

Halve the Brussel sprouts and steam over boiling water.

In a large mixing bowl, combine the cooked fish, Brussel sprouts and cauliflower "sauce." Gently mix and transfer to an oven safe dish.

Dot the top with roasted butternut squash, sprinkle with chopped pistachios and drizzle with extra virgin olive oil.

Cover with foil and bake for 30 minutes. Then, remove the foil and broil until golden brown.

For the Butternut Squash:

Preheat oven to 375ºF. While oven is preheating, remove rind from squash and cut into one-bite pieces. (Alternatively, you can often find pre-cut butternut squash in some grocery stores).

Drizzle squash with olive oil and sprinkle with salt. Bake until tender, about 15-20 minutes.

Oven Roasted Trout

Makes 4 servings

<u>Ingredients</u>

2 fresh rosemary sprigs
2 garlic cloves, minced
1 small shallot, finely diced
Salt and freshly ground white pepper, to taste
1 ½ lb new potatoes, peeled and thinly sliced
4 tbsp extra-virgin olive oil
2 tbsp unsalted butter, cut into small pieces
4 small trout fillets
Fresh parsley, for garnish

<u>Method</u>

Preheat oven to 375°F.

Finely chop the leaves of one rosemary sprig and combine with garlic and shallot in a small bowl. Add a liberal amount of salt and white pepper.

Place half the potato slices in rows along the bottom of a well-oiled baking dish, allowing the slices and rows to overlap slightly.

Evenly sprinkle one-third of the garlic-shallot mixture over the potatoes, drizzle with 1½ tbsp of olive oil and dot with 1 tbs of butter. Layer in the rest of the potato slices and top with one-third of the garlic-shallot mixture, 1 ½ tbsp of oil and the remaining butter.

Cover the dish and bake for 20 minutes. Uncover and continue baking until the potatoes are almost tender, about 20 minutes more.

Remove the dish from the oven. Place the fish evenly atop the potatoes. Drizzle with the remaining olive oil and sprinkle with the remaining garlic-shallot mixture. Place the other, whole rosemary sprig on top. Return to the oven and bake until the fillets are opaque, about 10 minutes. Let rest for 10 minutes, then serve.

CHAPTER 3 – COD HEARTED

"Listen, man. It's been over a week. You haven't found Tam, the mystery fish lady, and you need a date for your sister's wedding. Hear me out and just try Tindr. Everyone's doing it. It's not even a big deal." Kat pops a grape into her mouth.

"I don't know. What will people think?" Binh toys with the string on his tea bag. They are sitting in the window seat of a quaint cafe near Binh's accounting office. It's the kind of place that still uses lace doilies and smells like a favorite old book.

"They'll think you're looking for a date, which is true, and there's no shame in it. Just give me your phone. I'll set it all up." Kat lunges for Binh's phone and nearly knocks over his tea in the process.

"Watch it!" Binh exclaims.

Kat adroitly makes a series of taps and swipes on Binh's phone. "Now just to set a profile picture. Say cheese." The flash leaves Binh seeing stars. His eyes are closed in the photo.

"No. That won't do," says Kat. Seven photographs later, Kat is finally pleased with her work and hands the phone back to Binh. "There you go. All set up. It's really easy. Just swipe left if you're not interested and swipe right if you are."

Binh studies the phone. He gingerly swipes the screen a half dozen times. "This is silly," he says.

"It's not. Here, look." Kat leans across the table to peer at the phone.

"You've got your first match. Send her a message. Ask her to that new place that just opened on Market St. I know the owner. I can get you a table."

"I don't know what to say." Binh lays the phone, screen up, on the pastel patchwork tablecloth.

"Just tell her the truth. You're an accountant. A good job's a big turn-on, and you're looking for a date to your sister's wedding. Wanting to meet up with someone beforehand to make sure you get along. Or, y'know what. Just let me do it." Kat scoops the phone up again. She performs a few rapid motions and thrusts the phone back into Binh's hands. "There. You're getting dinner on Friday at 7:00. Wear your blue tie."

Binh sighs. "Okay. I guess."

"What about 'Thanks, Kat. I don't know what I'd do without you, Kat.'?" She pops another grape and grins.

* * *

Binh is sitting alone at a table for two near the bar. He stirs the ice in his water. He checks his phone for the third time. It reads 7:15. Fifteen minutes is nothing. Maybe she's stuck in traffic or took too long getting ready.

"Would you like to order an appetizer sir? Or perhaps I could bring you something to drink besides water?" The waiter is growing annoyed.

There's a two-hour wait to be seated tonight, and here this guy is, sipping water--alone--and checking his watch. Who does he think he is? He needs to learn when to cut his losses.

"Oh, no. Sorry to be a bother. Water is fine for now. She should be here any minute. Sorry. Again." Binh tucks his head and peers up from under his brow at the waiter. This guy has had it with me. I don't know what will be more embarrassing--being stood up or getting asked to leave.

"Okay, sir. Let me know if you need anything else." The waiter responds, mechanically, as he walks away.

The restaurant is crowded and loud. Stark white linens drape each table in the dim, moody light. Plush, hunter green carpets, not yet worn by foot traffic or stained by spills, help to dull the din of over-dinner conversation, bringing the noise level down to a dull roar. Golden sconces shine like fireflies on the dark matte and gloss relief wallpaper. A large, elaborate chandelier hangs from the high ceiling, over the large group table in the center of room.

At the table next to Binh, an older businessman laughs at his much younger date's joke. She leans over the table and dabs his face with a napkin. Giggling,

25

she reclines back in her own chair, reaches for her champagne, and wraps her slender fingers around the stem. Her long legs cross at the ankles, exposing a hint of red from her Louboutin heels.

Binh looks away from the couple, and back down at his phone. He opens the Tindr app and checks, yet again, to see if his date has sent a message confirming his suspicions that she's not coming. Nothing. He considers asking her if she's still coming or if she needs to reschedule.

"I'm at the restaurant. Will you be joining me?" No. Too formal. Binh deletes the message and starts over. "Hey, girl. Just wondering where you at. lol" Oh, God, no. That's not me at all.

Exasperated, Binh shuts off his phone and stuffs it in his pocket. He leaves a nice tip for his patient waiter and quietly leaves, hoping no one has noticed him.

Outside, in the dewy night air, Binh stands behind a pink-hued streetlamp and hails a cab. He rides in silence back to his loft. His phone doesn't make a peep.

Binh climbs the five flights of stairs and walks through his creaking door. Ginger greets him with a gentle meow.

"Hey, Ging. I think you might be the only girl for me. Let's get you some dinner." As he picks up Ginger's bowl and walks toward the pantry where he keeps the kibble, Binh's stomach growls.

"I guess I need some dinner, too, huh?" Binh says absently to Ginger as she nuzzles against him in anticipation of food. "I know. We'll have some comfort food. I'll make Ba's baked fish cakes."

Binh places Ginger's bowl back on the floor near the breakfast bar, then preheats the oven.

HERO RECIPE – Ba's Baked Cod Cakes

Makes 3-4 servings

<u>Ingredients</u>

1 lb. Cod, poached & flaked
¼ cup shallots, minced
¼ cup breadcrumbs
¼ cup cornmeal
2 eggs
1 tsp salt
½ tsp pepper
½ tsp honey

<u>Method</u>

Preheat oven to 400ºF.

Poach the cod, being careful not to overcook. Do not boil, because the fish will become too chewy.

Flake the cod with a fork, and combine all ingredients in a large mixing bowl.

Shape into patties, about 2-3 inches in diameter. The batter will be wet, but not runny.

Bake for 20 minutes at 400ºF.

Lemon Baked Cod

Makes 4 servings

<u>Ingredients</u>

3 tbsp lemon juice
3 tbsp butter, melted
1/4 cup all-purpose flour
1/2 tsp salt
1/4 tsp paprika
1/4 tsp cracked black pepper
4 6 oz cod fillets
2 tbsp minced fresh parsley
2 tsp lemon zest

<u>Method</u>

Preheat oven to 400° F.

Combine lemon juice and butter in a small bowl.

In a separate shallow bowl, mix flour and seasonings.

Dip fillets in lemon juice mixture, then in flour mixture. Coat both sides. Shake off excess.

Spray a 13 x 9 dish with cooking spray. Place fillets in the dish and drizzle with remaining lemon juice butter.

Bake for 15 minutes, or until fish flakes with a fork. Mix parsley & lemon zest and sprinkle over fish.

FISH TACOS

Makes 4 servings

<u>Ingredients</u>

½ red onion, thinly sliced
2 cloves garlic, minced
1 ½ cups red wine vinegar
¼ cup olive oil
1 ½ tsp red chili powder
1 ½ tsp dried oregano
½ tsp ground cumin
¼ cup fresh cilantro leaves, chopped, plus more for garnish
1 jalapeño, stemmed and chopped
1-pound cod, cut into 4 pieces
Salt
8 corn tortillas Mexican crema Pineapple Salsa
2 limes, quartered

<u>Method</u>

For The Onion:

In a small bowl, combine onion and red wine vinegar. There should be just enough to cover the onion completely. Allow to sit for at least 30 minutes, or up to 2 weeks.

For The Fish:

In a separate small bowl, mix together the olive oil, garlic, chili powder, oregano, cumin, chopped cilantro and jalapeño. Place the fish in a Ziploc bag and pour in the marinade. Shake the bag to fully coat the fish. Let marinate for at least 20 minutes.

Heat a nonstick sauté pan over medium-high heat. Place the marinated fish in the hot pan and season with salt. Cook for 4 minutes on the first side, flip, and cook for an additional 2 minutes.

Remove the pan from the heat. Flake the fish with fork and be sure to mix in all the marinade remaining in the pan. Taste and salt, if needed. Set aside.

For The Salsa:

Combine 2 diced fresh tomatoes, 1 diced medium onion, cilantro, 1 clove garlic, ½ cup chunk pineapple and 1 tsp salt into a food processor. Blend until combined, but still chunky.

To Serve:

Warm a small skillet over medium heat. Warm each tortilla, flipping once to heat both sides. Assemble the tacos. Scoop a heaping tsp of the fish onto two overlapping tortillas. Top with onions and cilantro. Serve with lime wedges, Mexican crema and pineapple salsa.

Asian Steamed Cod

Makes 2 servings

<u>Ingredients</u>

1" thick fresh cod steak
Fresh ginger
White pepper

For The Sauce:

1 tbsp light soy sauce
1 tsp sugar
1 tbsp water
1 tbsp rice cooking wine
1 tsp galangal (optional)

For The Garnish:

3 cloves garlic, finely chopped
1 tbsp peanut oil
1 tsp sesame oil
1 green onion, thinly sliced

<u>Method</u>

Place two slices of fresh ginger in a steamer and lay the fish on top.

Bring water to boil in a stock pot and place the bamboo steamer on top. Allow to steam for 7 minutes.

Heat all sauce ingredients in a medium saucepan.

In another pan, fry chopped garlic with peanut and sesame oil until golden brown. Remove fish from steamer and pour off any liquid that may have pooled on the fish. Add a dash of white pepper and pour the sauce over the fish.

Pour the hot garlic oil over fish, garnish with golden brown garlic and spring onions. Serve immediately!

CHAPTER 4 – WILL YOU MAHI ME?

It was a beautiful ceremony. A guest list as big as Binh's sister Chau's personality and colors as bright as her mind. Deep purples and vibrant blues draped the tables, chairs and rafters of the large reception hall. Now, Binh is seated at a circular table near the dais, watching the guests pour in.

Kat makes a beeline for Binh's table and plops down next to him, even cheerier than usual. The reason for this elation soon appears: Amy is following close behind. She perches gently in the high-backed chair next to Kat.

"I still can't believe you couldn't find a date," Kat says, half annoyed, half gently teasing. "I mean, when you fall off the horse, you have to get back on. One bad date and, bam, Binh gives up."

"Kat, don't," Amy says firmly, but compassionately. "Online dating isn't for everyone."

"Yeah. It definitely wasn't for me." Binh says. "That's no way to meet people. Plus, y'know, Tam. I can't stop thinking about her."

"Oh. Em. Gee. If I have to hear about Tam one more time..."

Amy cuts Kat off, "Stop it. Lay off him. Love is funny. We're proof."

She lays her head in the crook of Kat's shoulder and closes her eyes.

"Yeah, what's going on here, anyway?" Binh asks. The last he knew, Kat and Amy had called it quits.

"Well, like I said, love is funny." Amy rights herself and smiles.

"I ran into her at the shop, while I was getting fitted for this fabulous getup. Last minute, of course." Kat gestures to herself, swooping her arms up and down her torso and swerving her head with her characteristic sass.

"She asked if I was still her plus one to Chau's wedding. And you know how I love your sister..." Amy pipes up.

"Long story short, she said yes and I charmed her back into my life." Kat grins smugly. Amy playfully slapped her arm. "Oh, hush. It's just that being here, feeling all this love. I remembered how much I cared for Kat and how good the good times were."

Amy and Kat share a smile and gaze into each other's eyes with the intensity of new lovers.

"Well, I'm happy for you," Binh says, mustering all the positivity he could. "Maybe someday I'll have that for myself."

"Oh, shut up. You know you will," Kat says flippantly.

"Actually, I was going to tell you earlier, but then you said you didn't want to hear more about Tam. But there's been I development. I found out..." Binh couldn't finish his sentence. The appearance of the bride overshadows his announcement.

Chau is standing at their table in her wedding gown. "Thank you guys so much for coming!"

Chau beams at the group, making the rounds, hugging necks and kissing cheeks.

"You're such a beautiful bride!" "It was the most touching ceremony."

"I'm so proud of you, sis. You bagged a real good man." A chorus of compliments emanates from the table.

"Thank you. Thank you. They're about to serve dinner, then we'll cut the cake and the dancing will begin!" Chau gives a little wiggle and a wide grin spreads across her face. "Okay, anyway, I have, like, 300 people to hug. See you on the dance floor!"

As she saunters away, Chau's train trails behind her. Her dress is a spectacle. Even bustled, her train extends a good two feet behind her. Sleeveless with a sweetheart neck, the cut accentuates Chau's pronounced collar bones, and the corset cinched waist creates a dramatic contrast with her full, billowing skirt. The bodice is encrusted with rhinestones and accented in silver filigree. She's forgone the traditional lace veil for a glittering tiara. Chau shines like a star, and lights up every table she graces. A true picture of a stunning, modern bride.

"Were you saying something, Binh? About Tam?" Amy softly nudges.

"Yeah, actually, I found out where she works." Binh perks at the thought.

"So she's real! She's really real!" Kat exclaims with over-the-top zealousness. And then, "I'm starving."

Amy cuts her eyes at Kat. "So, back to Tam, where does she work, Binh? Are you going to go talk to her?"

"She's working the counter at the vintage boutique near the Starbucks on Fourth Street. I saw her through the window on my way to get my morning coffee, and I just about ran into a lady pushing a stroller."

"Ha!" Binh had Kat's attention again. "Okay, here's what you're gonna do..." Kat trailed off. Dinner has started to appear. "Do you smell that? I'm so hungry. I got the prime rib. You?"

"Mahi-mahi," Binh responds, dejectedly. Kat can't concentrate when she's hungry. I'll wait until after dinner and maybe we can stay on topic.

"Me, too. Mahi-mahi," Amy replies.

Kat chuckles. "Will you mahi me, Amy? C'mon. Let's get mahi-mahied. Ah. Here it comes!" A server clad all in black places a heavy plate in front of each guest at the table.

Amy groans. "Your puns are the worst. Now I remember why we broke up." Amy shoots Kat a coy smile.

"Hey. Wait until I'm done eating to pick on me. I'm hungry." Kat cuts into her meat, swabs it in her mashed potatoes, and takes a bite.

"Aaaaaah. So good."

The mahi-mahi is teriyaki glazed and served over a bed of rice with a side of grilled asparagus. Buttery in texture with balanced flavors that don't overpower the fish, the meal hits the spot and lifts Binh's spirits. There's nothing like good food to smooth the mood between friends, he thinks, looking up from his plate at the smiling faces surrounding him.

Once the plates are cleared away and Kat's blood sugar returns to normal levels, conversation around Tam and Binh resumes.

"Before you started shoveling food into your face, I think you were trying to help our friend Binh here with his love woes." Amy nudges Kat gently in the ribs.

"Oh. Yeah. Right. Okay. It's really simple." Kat folds her arms behind her head and leans back in her chair. "You go into the shop and talk to her."

"Wow. Amazing. I wish I would have thought of that," Binh chides.

"Just pretend you're looking for a gift for your mom or sister or other non-girlfriend person of the female persuasion. If she's not there, 'accidentally' leave some small possession behind, like a notebook or a pair of sunglasses. Then wait until you see her in the shop, go in, and inquire about the item. It's all about manufacturing an excuse to talk to her. Then just ask her out. The worst that can happen is she'll say no." Kat smirks, pleased with herself and her plan and her belly full of prime rib.

"That sounds like a good plan to me," Amy agrees. The women look at Binh for a response. With hesitation, he slowly says, "Okay...I'll give it a try.

HERO RECIPE: Mahi-Mahi In White Wine Herb Reduction

Makes 4 servings

<u>Ingredients</u>

1 lb mahi-mahi fillets
½ cup white wine
2 garlic cloves, minced
½ tsp salt
¼ tsp pepper
1 tsp tarragon
1 tsp marjoram
2 tbsp butter
1 tsp honey

<u>Method</u>

Salt and pepper the fish fillets.

Combine dry spices in a small ramekin.

Melt the butter in a deep pan over medium heat.

When butter begins to bubble, add the garlic and cook until fragrant.

Add the wine and honey. Reduce by half (about 5-7 minutes).

Place the fillets in the pan and simmer until done, about 15 minutes or until the internal temperature reaches 165°F.

Flip halfway through cooking and spoon the beurre blanc sauce over the fillets frequently as they cook.

Remove from heat, sprinkle with the spice blend and serve immediately.

Honey Lime Mahi-Mahi

Makes 4 servings

Ingredients

For the chili lime butter:

4 tbsp unsalted butter, room temperature
1 tsp salt
1 tsp honey
½ tsp chipotle powder
½ tsp chili powder zest from 2 limes

For the pan seared mahi-mahi:

4 6-oz wild caught mahi-mahi fillets
1 tbsp coconut oil
salt and pepper to taste

Method

Chili lime butter

In a small bowl, beat together all ingredients.

Heat a large skillet over medium high heat. Lightly salt and pepper the fillets.

Melt the coconut oil in the hot pan, and add the fillets.

Cook 5 minutes per side, or until golden brown and a meat thermometer reads an internal temperature of 145° F.

Plate the mahi-mahi and top with 1 tablespoon of chili lime butter. Serve warm with lime wedges.

GRILLED MAHI-MAHI

Makes 4 servings

<u>Ingredients</u>

4 medium mahi-mahi fillets

For the marinade:

2 tbsp extra virgin olive oil
2 tbsp fresh ginger, minced
1 clove garlic, minced
1 tbsp fresh lime juice
¼ cup soy sauce
2 tbsp honey
2 tbsp rice wine
One dried chili pepper, crushed
A pinch of star anise salt and pepper

<u>Method</u>

Mix all marinade ingredients in a Ziploc bag. Handle the bag until all ingredients are combined. Add the fish to the bag and refrigerate for at least 4 hours or overnight.

Lubricate the grill with nonstick cooking spray and heat to 475° F.

Grill fillets for 4 minutes on the first side, or until firm. Flip and cook another 2-3 minutes. Use a meat thermometer--you don't want to overcook your fish. The safe internal temperature for fish is 145° F.

BALSAMIC GLAZED MAHI-MAHI

Makes 4 servings

<u>Ingredients</u>

4 6 oz. Mahi-Mahi fillets
2 tbsp stone ground mustard
1 tsp extra virgin olive oil
3 tsp balsamic vinegar
2 tsp honey
1 tsp dry red wine

<u>Method</u>

Whisk wet ingredients together in a small bowl.

Place mahi-mahi in a Ziploc bag and pour marinade into the bag. Shake to coat. Refrigerate for at least 30 minutes.

Using a grill pan, cook until the internal temperature reaches 145° F, or about 4 minutes on each side.

CHAPTER 5 – SHE'S SWAI I SMILE

The sound of Binh's trainers on the pavement adds a rhythmic bass line to the cheery melody of the songbirds. Ever since he found out where Tam works, he's had a new morning routine: a 3-mile run through the park, followed by coffee and a danish at the Starbucks near the shop where Tam works. He reads the paper-- or rather, pretends to read the paper-- and waits with bated breath to see if she'll appear. He's seen her five times in the past two weeks and has yet to work up the nerve to follow through with Kat's plan.

Binh crosses the wooden bridge spanning the gently babbling creek. The flowers are in full bloom and the elm trees tout luscious crowns of green. A pink Dogwood sways gently in the breeze, releasing fragrant petals that flutter to the ground.

I'm going to do it today. I really am, Binh thinks to himself. He whispers Tam's name gently with each exhalation and pushes himself to hasten his pace. Today will be the day.

Run done, Binh jogs heavily to the park's water fountain and takes a long, cool drink. He hops around on his toes a bit, stretches his arms over his head and bends at the waist to place his hands on the ground, then walks to a nearby bench to finish his post-run stretches.

While he contorts in stretch, targeting his hamstrings--foot propped on the bench, leg bent, bowed over himself, eyes level with his knee--an elderly couple shuffles into his peripheral view.

The woman stoops over her walker and shuffles her slippered feet as she shambles merrily along. Her husband is at her side, one hand supporting her elbow and both eyes on her smiling face. As he helps her navigate the winding sidewalk, they whisper and giggle to each other like children. Her floral dress sways like the Dogwood and her arched back belies the youthful sparkle in her eyes. He tilts his head back and laughs deeply, his voice surprisingly full. The couple continues on their leisurely journey to the bench opposite Binh.

Binh continues his stretching as the couple moves within earshot. Is it eavesdropping if it's unavoidable? Binh asks himself.

"...remember the first time we came here?" He helps her settle onto the bench under a canopy of low-hanging Honey Locust branches.

"Oh, that was so long ago," she chuckles and continues, "I think... wasn't it during a school event? For a project? Yeah. Yeah, it was Arbor Day, I believe. We were here to clean up the park."

"That's right. We planted that tree over there," he says, motioning.
"We did?" she exclaims.

"Oh, I don't know," he admits. "I don't remember the first time we came here. I just wanted you to tell me a pretty story." He gazes into her full, bright eyes and a sly grin spreads across his face.

"Oh, you!" She gently taps him on the shoulder, scoffs and then laughs. Her whole body shakes with the gesture.

Binh stifles his own laughter and wraps up his stretches. I wonder how Mom and Dad are. I should give them a call. Maybe ask them for dinner. He collects his water bottle and sunglasses, pulls his phone from his arm holster and dials his mom's number as he begins his cool down walk near the front of the park.

"Hello? Binh? Is that you? This is your mother speaking." "Hi, yes, Mom, I know. I called you."
"Oh! Hi, Binh. What's going on?"

"I just finished my run in the park and I was wondering if you and Dad would like to get together for dinner tonight?"

"That sounds just lovely! What time would you like to come eat? I usually have dinner ready about five-thirty, quarter to six."

"That's nice, Mom, but I was thinking I could take you all out somewhere in the city."

"Nonsense. You'll come eat here with your father and me. We're having curry. Be here by 5:30 if you want it while it's hot. Love you, Binh. Your father says hi. See you tonight!"

Binh begins to when his phone begins beeping loudly in his ear. He pulls it away with from his head with a jump. His mother had already hung up. Well, I guess that's that, Binh sniggers and gives his head a little shake. Now's there's just one thing I have to do.

Binh puts his phone back in its holster, tucks his sunglasses into his shirt and stuffs his towel into the pocket in his running shorts. He breathes deeply and walks across the street to Tam's store.

* * *

Binh opens the door to the shop and is greeted by a spirited bell and a friendly "Hello, sir. Can I help you with something?"

The cordial voice is not Tam's. I don't know to be relieved or disappointed, Binh thinks. "Yes, hello. I'm looking for a small gift for my mother."

"Is it her birthday or is there a special occasion?" the perky young shop girl asks. Her smile is warm and genuine. She's roughly 5 inches shorter than Binh, plump in a pleasant way, with a short, pixie haircut that brings attention to her large, round eyes.

"Oh, no occasion. It's a just-because gift."

The shop girl's face softens. "Aw, how sweet. Your mother is lucky to have a son like you. Let me show you a few pieces from some local artists and jewelry makers that she might like."

Binh selects a jade comb with a jeweled cherry blossom adornment and is careful to accidentally leave his water bottle among the shop goods.

* * *

"Oh Binh, you're here!" His mother is waiting at the door when he arrives. She embraces him immediately, squeezing a little more than is necessary.

"Come. Sit. Dinner's almost ready. I told you we're having curry, right? Do you want tea?"

"Yes. Tea would be great. Here, mom. I got you a little something." Binh kisses his mother on the cheek and produces the comb from his jacket pocket. Freshened up from his run, Binh is now sporting a crisp pair of olive green khakis, an off-white polo and navy sports jacket. His mother always appreciates it when he looks presentable, as she would put it.

"Oh, you shouldn't have! Binh, it's lovely. Look, hon. Look what Binh brought me."

Binh's father sits at the head of the table, a few papers scattered in front of him. His glasses hang from his pronounced ears, resting halfway down the bridge of his nose. He looks up long enough to get a glimpse of the trinket in his wife's hands.

"That's nice dear," Binh's father replies and looks back at his paperwork.

"Your father's got it in his head that he's going to buy a boat. Nonsense. But it keeps him busy and out of my hair, so I let him have his little fantasy." Binh's mother talks as she enters the kitchen and returns with a steaming bowl of curry. "Get the rice would you?"

Once the food is on the table and the family is settled around it, Binh's mother starts in on him. "So, tell me about this girl you're courting."

Binh freezes, a forkful of curry suspended in midair. "Courting is a bit of an overstatement. Right now it feels more like light stalking. I haven't had the courage to ask her out yet. But I have a plan."

"Well, you'd better hurry up," his mother replies, wiping her mouth. "And besides, any girl would be lucky to have you."

"Thanks, Mom." Binh finishes his bite of curry. *Just like when I was a kid. His mother's cooking has a way of setting the world right again.*

HERO RECIPE: Almost Homemade Fish Curry

Makes 5-6 servings

<u>Ingredients</u>

1 lb. swai, chopped
3 small red skin potatoes
1 onion, halved and sliced
½ bunch kale, chopped
¼ cup chives, chopped
1 can lite coconut milk
1 can regular coconut milk
1 ½ tbsp red curry paste (available in most International aisles or Asian markets)
1 tbsp peanut oil
1 cup saffron rice, cooked
Salt to taste
Sour Cream or yogurt (optional)

<u>Method</u>

Heat stock pot over medium heat. Once hot, add peanut oil and stir in red curry paste and lite coconut milk.

Add potatoes and bring to a boil.

Add swai, onion, kale and regular coconut milk. Cook until vegetables soften.

Season with salt to taste. Serve over rice and garnish with chives and sour cream or yogurt, if desired.

Baked Swai

Makes 4 servings

<u>Ingredients</u>

4 6 oz. Swai fillets Butter, chilled Turmeric
Paprika
Salt & pepper

<u>Method</u>

Preheat the oven to 350ºF.

While the oven preheats, rub the fillets with turmeric and allow to sit.

Once the oven has preheated, place the fillets in a lightly greased casserole dish. Sprinkle the fillets with salt, pepper and paprika.

Baked for 15-20 minutes or until fish is flaky. Serve immediately with lemon.

Dijon Swai

Makes 4 servings

Ingredients

4 6 oz swai fillets
2 eggs, beaten
3 tbsp Parmesan cheese
Zest of one lemon
1 tbsp Dijon mustard
1 tsp horseradish
¼ cup panko
2 tsp butter, melted

Method

Preheat oven to 425ºF and line a baking sheet with parchment paper or use a silicon mat.

Beat the eggs until frothy. Combine with 2 tbsp Parmesan cheese, lemon juice, Dijon mustard and horseradish.

Spread the mixture over the fillets.

In a small bowl, stir together panko, butter and the other tbsp of Parmesan. Sprinkle over the fish.

Bake for 15-20 minutes or until fish easily flakes and breadcrumb topping is golden brown.

SWAI STIR FRY

Makes 3-4 servings

<u>Ingredients</u>

1 lb swai fillets
2 bags frozen stir fry vegetables (½ sliced onion, 1 sliced green bell pepper, 1 sliced red bell pepper, snap peas)
2 tbsp Peanut oil
½ tsp Sesame oil
2 tbsp Soy sauce
1 clove garlic, minced
1 in. fresh ginger, minced
1 tbsp Chinese Five Spice mix (anise, clove, cinnamon, chili powder, fennel seed)
1 cup rice (white or brown), cooked according to package directions

<u>Method</u>

Cut the swai into two-bite chunks. Set aside. Heat the oils until hot over medium-high heat.

Add the frozen vegetables, garlic and ginger; stir often until onions are translucent. Add the fish, soy sauce and spices.

Cook, stirring often, until fish is white and flaky. Serve immediately over rice.

CHAPTER 6 – LOST AND FLOUNDER

The next day Binh stakes out Tam's shop from the Starbucks on the corner. Sitting at the patio table farthest from the building, Binh can just peer through the window of the shop--if he cranes his neck. He wads up a napkin and nonchalantly walks to the trash can nearer the shop's entrance.

She's there in all her dazzling glory. Standing behind the counter, totally oblivious to the fact that Binh even exists. She's laughing at a customer's joke. She flips her hair behind her shoulder with one elegant sweep of her slender arm.

I can do this. Binh rallies every drop of courage and confidence he can find within himself. He balls his fists, stands up straight and puts one foot in front of the other. His hand is on the door now. He pushes. The doorbell rings. Tam looks up and sees Binh for the very first time.

"Good afternoon. May I help you find something?"

"Actually, I, uh..." Binh clears his throat. "I was in here yesterday.

Another girl helped me buy a gift for my mom," Why did I add that part? I sound like a child or like I'm complaining about the stuff she sells. I'm so stupid, "and, uh, I left my water bottle behind. I was hoping maybe it was still here?" Binh's voice jumps higher in pitch than he would have liked, and he feels the last syllable he squeaked out hanging awkwardly in the air.

"Oh! Were you the one who bought the jade comb? I always loved that piece. You have excellent taste." Tam's eyes turn to radiant half moons as she smiles.

Is she flirting with me or just doing her job? Binh wonders. Probably just doing her job. But a man can dream.

"If you'll follow me to the counter, I'll check the lost and found for you." Tam gives Binh one more quick smile and turns. She weaves effortlessly through the cramped boutique without disturbing a single item. Binh blunders through the tiny aisle, knocking askew leather mini skirts, feathered cardigans and busily patterned A-line dresses, and releasing tiny motes and floral, musty scents into the air.

Tam ducks out of view and rummages under the counter. She re-emerges with a smirk on her face. Leaning across the counter, forearms extended, almost touching Binh, she playfully informs him, "Yes. We do have a bottle back here. But you'll have to ask me out for lunch if you want to get it back."

Binh nearly trips over his jaw. He reaches out and steadies himself with the counter. Did that just happen? All these weeks of anxiety and agony and I could have just waltzed in here and this would have happened. This cannot be real.

"I.. uh, I. Um. Are you sure..." Binh stammers. "Uh, yeah. Lunch. That is a meal people have together. And you and I can have it, I mean, lunch, together."

Tam giggles. "How about a picnic? It's perfect picnic weather. I'm off tomorrow. Meet you at noon in Centre Park? In front of the fountain?" She dangles the water bottle inches from the counter's top.

"Yes!" Binh exclaims. A shopper near the front of the store swivels her head and jumps at the sudden sound. "I mean, uh, yeah. I could do that." Smooth, Binh chides himself.

"Okay," Tam sets the bottle down slowly and slides it across the counter to Binh. "I guess I'll see you then. My name's Tam."

"I'm Binh." He reaches out to reclaim his bottle. His hand grazes Tam's, and she doesn't pull away.

"See you tomorrow, Binh." Tam pronounces his name slowly, rolling each sound around in her mouth before letting it escape from her barely parted lips.

*   *   *

"Oh. Em. Gee. I literally cannot even compete with that," Kat bursts into surprised laughter.

"That is the coolest thing to ever happen to you since the time that old lady mistook you for John Cho from Harold and Kumar and wouldn't leave you alone until you signed an autograph for her grandson."

"Thanks, Kat. Your empathy and compassion truly knows no bounds," Binh lays the sarcasm on thick.

"But, seriously, tho. This is cause for celebration, don't you think?" "You think everything is cause for celebration."

"Well it is! Life is great! Let Amy and I take you to Verretti's for dinner. Our treat. You deserve it, lady killer." Kat bellows more laughter on the other end of the phone.

"Aahh. You know I can't resist Italian food."

"I know you like the back of my hand. I'll make reservations. How does 7 sound?"

"Sounds great, Kat. Give Amy my love."

HERO RECIPE: Flounder Mediterranean

Makes 3-4 servings

<u>Ingredients</u>

1 lb flounder fillets
15-20 grape tomatoes
2 tbsp olive oil
1 shallot, chopped
1 clove garlic, chopped
½ tsp basil
½ tsp oregano
¼ cup white wine
¼ cup capers
Juice of ½ lemon
3 tbsp Parmesan cheese

<u>Method</u>

Preheat the oven to 425°F.

While the oven is preheating, half and skin your tomatoes by quickly boiling and soaking in ice water. They should then easily peel off.

Heat the olive oil in a large skillet over medium heat. Add the shallot and garlic. Cook for 2 minutes or until fragrant.

Add the tomatoes, basil and oregano. Cook until the tomatoes are tender.

Stir in the capers, wine and lemon juice. Lower heat, mix in Parmesan cheese and reduce to a thick sauce.

Place flounder in a shallow baking dish and top with sauce. Cook 10-15 minutes, or until fish easily flakes with a fork.

Baked Flounder

Makes 4 servings

<u>Ingredients</u>

4 6 oz flounder fillets
1 tbs lemon juice
Zest from one lemon
2 tsp cracked peppercorns
½ tsp salt
2 garlic cloves, minced

<u>Method</u>

Preheat oven to 400ºF.

Place fillets on a greased baking sheet.

Combine lemon juice, zest, peppercorns, salt and garlic. Spread over the fillets. Bake for 10 minutes.

STUFFED FLOUNDER

Makes 4 servings

<u>Ingredients</u>

4 8 oz flounder fillets
1 cup crabmeat, flaked
1 tbsp green bell pepper, minced
1 tbsp onion, minced
¼ tsp salt
¼ tsp white pepper
Paprika
¼ cup panko or breadcrumbs
1 egg
1 tbsp mayonnaise
2 tbsp butter or margarine, melted

<u>Method</u>

Preheat oven to 400°F.

Place flounder fillets in a greased casserole dish. Brush with melted butter.

Combine crab meat, bell pepper, onion, salt, white pepper, panko, mayonnaise and egg. Spoon crab mixture onto fillets and fold fish over the crab mixture. Brush with melted butter.

Sprinkle with paprika.

Bake for 20-25 minutes until bubbly.

OVEN POACHED FLOUNDER

Makes 4 servings

<u>Ingredients</u>

4 6 oz flounder fillets, cut thin
⅓ cup extra virgin olive oil
3 garlic cloves, minced
1 sprig fresh thyme per fillet
White pepper
Salt
Lemon wedges

<u>Method</u>

Preheat oven to 375°F. Place flounder in a greased casserole dish.

Combine olive oil and garlic and pour over the fillets. Add one sprig of thyme to each. Sprinkle with salt and white pepper.

Bake for 15 minutes. Serve with lemon wedges.

CHAPTER 7 – NO OTHER FISH IN THE SEA

What to cook? What to cook? Binh opens and closes every cabinet in his kitchen at least twice, judging each to hold nothing more than disappointment. Why is this so hard? Ugh!. He gravitates toward the refrigerator, swings the door wide and nearly climbs inside.

Something healthy, but not too simple. Something portable that doesn't need a fancy presentation. Something that says, 'Hey, I'm sensible, but not too boring.' Tofu, no. Too bland. Not today, bacon. You go right back in that drawer. Ah! Tilapia. Yes, you will do nicely. Hey there, Spinach. Hello, cilantro! Looks like it's kedgeree for me.

Binh removes ingredients from the refrigerator and collects them neatly on the countertop. This will be great. Tasty at any temperature, filling but not too heavy. I hope Tam likes Sriracha.

*   *   *

Binh spreads a blanket under an old maple tree near the fountain in Centre Park. He unpacks his wicker basket--a gingham-lined one with a flip lid that he had borrowed from Amy at her insistence. Inside, he's stowed the tilapia kedgeree, a travel-sized bottle of Sriracha, plastic plates and utensils, a few bottles of Orangina, chocolate-covered strawberries for dessert and a single pink rose for Tam.

He sits atop the blanket next to the picnic spread and waits. And fidgets. And smoothes and re-smoothes the blanket. And checks his watch. 12:05. Please do not let me get stood up again. I don't think my ego could take it.

As that very thought leaves his head, Binh spies Tam walking toward the fountain to meet him. She's dressed in cream lace leggings and a simple coral pink shift dress that's belted at the waist. A lightweight open-knit shawl complements her leggings and accentuates her petite frame. On her feet are simple leather and hempen sandals with a modest wedge heel.

Binh leaps to his feet at the sight of her. He makes a conscious effort to keep from running out to greet her.

"Hi, Tam! It's me, Binh, from the other day." He winces as the words come out of his mouth. Tam giggles.

"I remember you, silly." She reaches out and playfully hits Binh's shoulder. "Yeah, of course you do. Sorry. Sometimes words just come out of my mouth before I think about it. Anyway, I've got a picnic set up under the tree there if you're hungry." Binh rubs the back of his neck and looks at the ground and then back to Tam as he talks. *I should just stop talking all together. What is wrong with me?*

The couple proceeds up the slight hill to the picnic Binh has laid out.

"Oh, this looks great! Chocolate strawberries are my favorite! Good thing I'm the eat-dessert-first type." Tam grins and selects a large, juicy berry from the bunch. Her lips wrap delicately around the fruit. Her shoulders heave and soften. She releases a small sigh. "So good." Her eyes shine and smile when she looks at Binh.

"So, tell me about yourself. All I know is that your name's Binh, you love your mom and you lose water bottles." Tam eats another strawberry.

"Ha. Well, I'm an accountant and a pescatarian and I like to play ultimate frisbee. Uh, my family is first generation Vietnamese. We were some of those refugee boat people. I was a little 6 year-old when we landed here. My favorite color is orange. Like, that pinkish burnt orange of wheat in the sunset light." *Why am I stammering on and on? I must sound like a freak...*

"Wow. And you're a poet, too."

"Hardly. What about you? Do you like working in the shop? Are you in school?" Binh knows she's in art school, but he doesn't want to let her know that he knows. *Don't let on that you're basically a stalker,* he thinks to himself.

"Yeah, the shop is fine, I guess. But I really want to be a sculptor. I'm in art school at the University, but they don't offer the specialty I want to go into." Tam's gaze fades into the distance. "Anyway. What's to eat?"

"Oh, yeah. I made kedgeree. Here let me get you some." Binh prepares Tam's lunch and gazes into her eyes as he passes her a plate. "But I still want to know more about you. What are you into?"

"Well," Tam takes a bite, "This is really good! Uh, mm, okay. I like acoustic music, like singer/songwriter kind of stuff, I'm obviously a sucker for a good museum. I like sculpting, duh. I like getting the clay and plaster under my fingers and stuck in my hair. It really makes you feel like you're doing something real, y'know? Um. I like to take candid photos of people on the street and in the subways, just living their life in a pure, raw way. I think my dad's disappointed in me. He's a banker and he was cursed with this free spirit creative daughter. He says I get it from my mother. But I wouldn't know. She died when I was still just a baby. Dad raised me all on his own, with the help of his mom, my Ba-Ba. He says that's why I'm not lady-like enough, but I think that, because I'm a lady, whatever I am is lady-like. He says that's another thing I get from my mother--bullheadedness."

She tosses her head back and laughs. "Almost makes me wonder what he saw in her that he doesn't see in me."

Tam stares off into space again, lost in her own thoughts. "But, there you have it. My whole life story in a nutshell. Dead mom, overbearing dad, silly dreams of making it as a starving artist. Once you get me going, I can really go, huh?"

"Your dreams aren't silly. You should always follow what makes you happy and fulfills you. And I like hearing about you. I like hearing about your dreams."

"Aw. That's maybe the sweetest thing anyone has ever said to me. So, Mr. Accountant. Does accounting 'fulfill' you?" Tam asks with a coquettish lilt to her voice.

"In a way, yes. I'm in private practice, so I have lots of flexibility. But I also really have to crunch during tax season, so the ebb and flow of workload can be stressful. And it's nice, because I have several big-ticket clients, so I can take on pro bono clients--like nonprofits and stuff--and feel like I'm really helping people."

"That is nice that you can help people who need it." Tam twirls the ends of her hair. "I wish sometimes that I had pursued something more practical. Something people actually need. But I didn't. And here I am. Leaving for Paris in two weeks on a wild goose chase. Or, at least, that's what my father would say. But...yeah..I guess he's a little bit right. I mean, it is kind of a big deal--uprooting and going to a new country and all."

Binh's heart sinks to his knees. She's leaving for Paris?! Yup. That sounds about right, doesn't? This is exactly the kind of thing that would happen to you. Wait until Kat hears this.

"Uh, whaa. Paris? Paris. I've heard Paris is nice this time of year. So, that should be fun. For you." She's going to goddamn Paris. "I guess. I just wish I would have asked you out sooner."

"What d'you mean? I asked you out, silly," Tam leans her back against Binh's right shoulder and arm."

"Yeah, but. I mean, I'd been trying to work up the nerve to ask you out for about three weeks now." Binh says and tentatively strokes Tam's hair with his left hand.

She sits up and turns to look at him. "Aw. Well, you should have. I had noticed you getting Starbucks the past couple weeks and I thought you were cute."

Tam drops her head like a too-heavy flower on a delicate stem and peers up at Binh. "But I guess it could have made my leaving harder."

"Well, you'll at least have to let me make you dinner before you go."

"Judging from your kedgeree, I think I'll have to agree."

"Was that a pun? That was terrible. Maybe I'll rescind my offer."

"Oh, don't do that." Tam places her hand on Binh's chest and leans in for a kiss.

HERO RECIPE: Picnic Kedgeree

Makes 2-3 servings

<u>Ingredients</u>

1 cup rice, cooked according to package directions
½ lb leftover fish, any variety
1 tbsp butter
1 cup spinach, stemmed and roughly chopped
½ cup green onions, chopped
2 tsp curry paste, your choice (available in most International sections or Asian markets)
1 dried red chili, crushed
1 handful parsley, chopped
½ lemon, juiced
2 hard-boiled eggs (optional)

<u>Method</u>

Melt the butter in a large, deep pan. Saute the chopped green onions until tender over medium heat.

Add the curry paste and dried chili. Stir and cook for about a minute.

Add the fish, cooked rice and spinach. Cook on high heat for 5 minutes, stirring frequently, then stir in the parsley and lemon juice.

Shell and half the eggs, if using, then place on top of the kedgeree and serve.

FISH SOUP

Makes 3-4 servings

<u>Ingredients</u>

1 lb leftover fish cut into 2 in. pieces
1 can crushed tomatoes (14 oz)
1 can clam juice (8 oz) or seafood/fish stock
6 tbsp olive oil
1 medium onion, diced
1 small bell pepper, diced
4 garlic cloves, minced
⅔ cup fresh cilantro, chopped
½ cup white wine
½ tsp Sriracha
Salt & pepper

<u>Method</u>

Heat olive oil in a stock pot over medium-high heat.

Saute onions and green pepper until onions are translucent. Add garlic and cilantro; cook for 2 minutes.

Add tomatoes; cook gently for 10 minutes.

Stir in clam juice, white fine, Sriracha and fish. Allow to simmer for 5 minutes. Salt and pepper to taste.

FISH QUINOA SALAD

Makes 2-3 servings

<u>Ingredients</u>

1 lb leftover fish
Quinoa, cooked according to package directions
10-12 cherry tomatoes, halved
3 tbsp chopped green onion
½ red onion, sliced
½ cup lime juice
¼ fresh cilantro, chopped
¼ cup raisins
2 tsp extra virgin olive oil
1 avocado, sliced
Salt & pepper

<u>Method</u>

Combine tomatoes, green and red onion, lime juice, cilantro, raisins and olive oil with cooked quinoa.

Top with warmed leftover fish and avocado. Serve immediately.

POSEIDON'S PASTA

Makes 2-3 servings

<u>Ingredients</u>

½ lb leftover fish
½ lb angel hair pasta
2 tbsp extra virgin olive oil
3 cloves garlic, minced
½ tsp salt
½ tsp coriander
1 lemon, juiced and zested Fresh dill, chopped Cracked black pepper

<u>Method</u>

Boil 6 quarts salted water. Cook pasta as per directions on bag.

In a fryer pan, heat olive oil over medium heat. Once hot, add lemon zest, coriander, and garlic. Stir for 30 seconds until aromatic.

Add fish, lemon juice, salt and ½ cup of pasta water to pan.

Drain pasta and combine with fish and sauce.

Sprinkle fresh dill and pepper on top and serve immediately.

ASIAN FISH PASTA

Makes 2-3 servings

<u>Ingredients</u>

1 lb leftover fish
½ lb wide rice noodles
2 tbsp lemon juice
2 tbsp lime juice
2 tbsp soy sauce
½ tsp fresh ginger, minced
1 tsp sesame oil
1 tsp brown sugar
1 scallion, diced
½ cup cilantro, chopped
½ cup shredded carrots
½ tsp anise
½ tsp cinnamon

<u>Method</u>

Soak rice noodles and cook according to directions on package.

Combine citrus juices, soy sauce, sesame oil and brown sugar in a medium bowl. Whisk to combine.

Add remaining ingredients and cooked pasta to mixture. Toss to coat. Serve immediately or refrigerate and serve chilled.

CHAPTER 8 – SOLE LONG, MY DEAR

"Ooooh, smells good. What's on the menu, gourmand?" Tam lets Binh help her with her coat as she enters his loft.

Binh hangs her lemon yellow, cinched-waist rain jacket on a rack near the door. The scent of her perfume mixed with rainwater is like sunshine on Binh's face.

"Sole Meuniere. I thought it was appropriate for a send-off to ol' Paree."

"You are so thoughtful. I wish I could bring you along to pamper and spoil me," Tam says with a wink.

Yes, in a heartbeat, Binh wants to blurt. "Hey, well, art school doesn't last forever, and I'm sure I'll still be around somewhere, thinking about stuff. When you get back."

"If I get back," Tams informs him. "I mean, that's where the scene is. You can't do what I do and be successful just anywhere. It's more than a career. It's a lifestyle."

"Just, y'know, trying to be positive. A spoonful of sugar, y'know?" Binh says.

"Yeah. Yeah, you're right. Let's just have a good time and eat this fancy French dinner you've made and be happy we had a happy two weeks." Tam kisses Binh on the cheek.

"I don't know how fancy it is, but it's just about ready. So I guess you can be the judge." Binh turns and steps into the kitchen to retrieve the dish from the oven. Tam walks further into his loft and turns her head from side to side, looking the place over.

"Nice little setup you have here. Accounting must be good to you." Tam turns the chair nearest the fireplace to face the kitchen and situates herself on it.

"It hasn't been bad." Binh lays a potholder on the breakfast bar and sets the dish atop it. "It's ready. I'll get some plates and silverware while it cools. Wine? I have a nice Pinot Grigio chilled."

"Wine would be great. Thanks."

*　　*　　*

The next morning, Tam lies sleeping in the crook of Binh's arm. The sun is trickling through the spaces between the Roman blinds, illuminating the strands of Tam's hair and adding depth to the shadows cast on the sheets from her body as it rises and falls with her gentle breaths. Binh kisses the top of her head and takes in the smell of her.

One last time, Binh thinks with a sigh.

Tam stirs. "Good morning, Binh." She rolls toward him and kisses his chest. "What time is it? My flight leaves at two."

"It's just now nine. You can go back to sleep if you want. I'll wake you." Binh hugs her against him.

"No. I want to make you breakfast. You're not the only one who can cook," Tam says, rolling out of bed and into the timid morning light. She is wearing white knee socks and one of Binh's old t-shirts. It comes down halfway to her knees, glancing off her small, well-rounded buttocks.

Tam prepares a simple breakfast of scrambled eggs, almost burnt bacon and half-toasted English muffins. Maybe I am the only one who can cook, Binh smirks to himself.

*　　*　　*

Tam embraces Binh as tightly as her slender frame will allow. They are standing near the security checkpoint at the airport. Tam is even shorter with her shoes off.

"Well, I guess this is goodbye," Tam says as she pulls away.

"I guess so. It was good getting to know you, Tam," Binh says with a catch in his throat.

"It was good getting to know you, Binh." Tam stands on her tiptoes, stretches upward and gives Binh one last kiss. "I'll always remember you when I eat Sole Meuniere."

"I'll always think of you, always." Binh wraps his hands around her upper arms and kisses her forehead. Tam turns makes her way through the checkpoints. After she recollects her belongings and puts her shoes and belt back on, she looks behind her and blows Binh a kiss. Then, with a wave, she's gone.

As Binh drives away from the airport, he wonders if he will ever see Tam again or will love always elude him.

HERO RECIPE: Sole Meunierette

Makes 2-3 servings

<u>Ingredients</u>

1 lb sole fillets
½ cup all purpose flour
1 tbsp butter
2 tbsp oil
1 tbsp lemon juice
Italian parsley, chopped
Salt & pepper

<u>Method</u>

Rinse fish fillets and pat dry. Sprinkle both sides with salt and pepper.

Dredge fillets in flour and set aside. Heat oil in large skillet on medium-high until hot. Add butter and swirl pan to coat.

Place fish in skillet and cook for 2 minutes on both sides. Use caution when turning; sole is a delicate fish. When done, remove to a heated plate.

Sprinkle with parsley and squirt with lemon juice. Serve immediately.

About The Author

Dr. Duc Vuong is an internationally renowned bariatric surgeon, who is the world's leading expert in education for the bariatric patient.

His intensive educational system has garnered attention from multiple institutions and medical societies. His passion in life is to fill the shortage of educational resources between patients and weight loss surgeons.

Although trained in Western medicine, he blends traditional Eastern teachings with the latest in science and technology. Dr. Vuong was featured in TLC's hit show, 900 Pound Man: Race Against Time, and is currently working on his own weekly television show.

Visit Dr. Duc Vuong at

www.SleeveAcademy.com

to learn more.

Other Books by Dr. Duc Vuong

Meditate to Lose Weight: A Guide For A Slimmer Healthier You

Healthy Eating on a Budget: A How-To Guide

Eating Healthy for Kids: A How-To Guide

Healthy Green Smoothies: 50 Easy Recipes That Will Change Your Life

Big-Ass Salads: 31 Easy Recipes For Your Healthy Month

Weight Loss Surgery Success: Dr. V's A-Z Steps For Losing Weight And Gaining Enlightenment

The Ultimate Gastric Sleeve Success: A Practical Patient Guide

Lap-Band Rescue: Revisit. Rethink. Revise.

Duc-It-Up: 366 Tips To Improve Your Life

Leave Me a Review!

If you enjoyed this book or found it useful, please take a moment to leave a review on Amazon. I'm always interested in learning what you like, think and want. I read all the reviews personally.

Thank you for your support!

Made in the USA
San Bernardino, CA
13 June 2018